SURVIVING TUBEROUS SCLEROSIS

Beginners Comprehensive Approach To Combating & Managing Tuberous Sclerosis Outbreak Effectively

Nuel Nenji

Table of Contents

Introductory

Tuberous sclerosis, also referred to as tuberous sclerosis complex (TSC), is an uncommon genetic disorder that can affect multiple organ systems. It is characterized by the development of benign tumors, or hamartomas, in a number of organs, including the brain, epidermis, kidneys, heart, eyes, and lungs.

These tumors are composed of abnormal cells that proliferate and divide uncontrollably, but they are typically benign and do not disseminate to other organs.

Mutations in the TSC1 or TSC2 genes, which regulate cell growth and proliferation, cause tuberous sclerosis. When these genes are mutated, they cease to function properly, resulting in the growth of malignancies in the affected organs.

Signs and symptoms of tuberous sclerosis can differ greatly from individual to individual and may include:

• Common skin manifestations include facial skin growths known as facial angiofibromas, hypomelanotic macules (light-colored regions), and fibrous skin plaques.

• Brain involvement: Tuberous sclerosis frequently affects the brain, causing cortical tubers, subependymal nodules, and subependymal giant cell astrocytomas to develop. These cerebral anomalies can result in convulsions, developmental delays, intellectual disabilities, and behavioral issues.

• Renal involvement: Renal angiomyolipomas, which are benign kidney tumors, may develop and produce pain, bleeding, or impairment of kidney function.

• Cardiac involvement: Cardiac rhabdomyomas, or heart tumors, are possible and may result in arrhythmias or other cardiac complications.

• Eye abnormalities: Retinal hamartomas and other eye conditions can occur and have the potential to impair vision.

Diagnostic criteria for tuberous sclerosis consist of clinical symptoms and genetic testing to identify mutations in the TSC1 or TSC2 genes. The treatment options for tuberous sclerosis seek to manage and alleviate the disorder's particular symptoms and complications.

These may include medications to control seizures, when necessary, surgical removal of lesions, and therapies to address developmental and behavioral difficulties.

Since tuberous sclerosis is a genetic disorder, it can be inherited from a parent who possesses a mutated TSC1 or TSC2 gene, but it can also arise spontaneously in individuals without a family history of the condition.

Affected individuals and their families are frequently advised to seek genetic counseling in order to better understand the risks of transmitting the condition to future generations and to make informed decisions about family planning. Tuberous sclerosis patients can substantially improve their quality of life through early diagnosis and intervention.

CHAPTER ONE
Prevalence And Population

Tuberous sclerosis (TSC) is a relatively uncommon genetic disorder with variable prevalence across populations.

It is estimated to affect between 1 in 6,000 and 1 in 10,000 births worldwide. However, certain subpopulations or geographic regions may have a higher prevalence.

Key aspects of the prevalence and demographics of tuberous sclerosis include the following.

• TSC affects both males and females in equal measure.

• There may be differences in the prevalence of TSC among various ethnic groups. Some studies indicate that it may be more prevalent in certain populations, such as those of Ashkenazi Jewish descent.

• Mutations in the TSC1 or TSC2 Genes: TSC is caused by mutations in these genes. Variable mutations and severity can result in a wide variety of clinical manifestations.

• TSC can be diagnosed at any age, ranging from infancy to maturity. Some individuals with subtle symptoms may not be diagnosed until later in life, whereas others with more severe manifestations may be diagnosed during infancy or childhood.

• Family History: TSC can occur sporadically in individuals with no family history of the disorder due to a new (de novo) mutation. In other instances, the disorder may be inherited from a parent with a mutated TSC1 or TSC2 gene.

• The severity of TSC symptoms can differ considerably between affected individuals. Some may have benign forms of the disorder with few or no discernible symptoms, whereas others may face more serious health issues.

• Neurological Involvement Neurological symptoms, such as epileptic seizures and cognitive deficits, are among the most prevalent and potentially severe manifestations of TSC.

• Skin Manifestations: Skin abnormalities, such as facial angiofibromas and hypomelanotic macules, are frequently early indications of TSC and are observed in a substantial proportion of affected individuals.

• Renal and Cardiac Involvement: Although less common, renal angiomyolipomas and cardiac rhabdomyomas are also significant clinical features of TSC.

Given the variable nature of TSC and the vast array of possible symptoms, demographics and prevalence can be affected by factors such as access to healthcare and the availability of diagnostic instruments. Early diagnosis and treatment of TSC are essential for enhancing patient outcomes and quality of life.

Importantly, ongoing research and advances in genetic testing have enhanced our understanding of TSC, and healthcare providers continue to refine diagnostic and treatment criteria for this complex disorder.

Individuals and families affected by TSC are frequently advised to seek genetic counseling in order to assess the risk of passing the condition on to future generations and to receive information and support.

Factors And Genes

Tuberous sclerosis (TSC) is caused by mutations in one of two genes: TSC1 (hamartin) and TSC2 (tuberin). These genes are responsible for regulating cell proliferation and growth. When mutations in either TSC1 or TSC2 occur, the normal control mechanisms are disrupted, leading to the development of benign tumors or hamartomas in various organs and tissues. Here are the main genetic and causative details of tuberous sclerosis:

• TSC is an autosomal dominant genetic disorder, meaning that an affected individual has a 50 percent chance of passing the mutated gene to each of their offspring. However, TSC frequently originates as a result of de novo mutations, which occur as a result of a new genetic change in an affected individual without a family history of the disorder.

• Mutations in the TSC1 gene, which is located on chromosome 9, are the cause of TSC in some individuals. This gene encodes the protein hamartin, which regulates the proliferation and division of cells.

• Mutations in the TSC2 gene, which is located on chromosome 16, are the most prevalent cause of TSC. Tuberin, which is encoded by the TSC2 gene, regulates cell growth and proliferation. Typically, mutations in the TSC2 gene exacerbate the severity of the disorder's symptoms.

• Two-Hit Hypothesis: The "two-hit" hypothesis is frequently used to describe TSC. Individuals inherit one mutated copy of either the TSC1 or TSC2 gene from a parent, according to this theory. The second impact, or mutation, spontaneously occurs in the other copy of the gene in certain body cells. This "second hit" results in the formation of tumors or hamartomas in those particular cells.

• Mosaicism: TSC can exhibit a mosaic pattern in which some cells in the body contain two copies of the mutated TSC1 or TSC2 gene while others do not. The severity and distribution of symptoms in affected individuals may be affected by the extent and location of mosaicism.

• Variability of Symptoms: The wide variety of TSC symptoms and organ involvement is partially attributable to the variable nature of genetic mutations, including the specific type of mutation and its location within the TSC1 or TSC2 gene. In addition, the proportion of cells with the second impact mutation can vary between affected individuals, resulting in varying clinical manifestations.

Notably, genetic testing can diagnose TSC and identify mutations in the TSC1 or TSC2 genes. Individuals and families affected by TSC should seek genetic counseling to learn about genetic risks, inheritance patterns, and family planning options.

In addition, ongoing research into the genetic basis of TSC continues to increase our understanding of the disorder and may one day lead to better treatments.

CHAPTER TWO
Observable Symptoms

Tuberous sclerosis (TSC) is a genetic disorder that can affect multiple organs and bodily systems. The signs and symptoms of TSC can vary greatly between affected individuals, and not everyone will exhibit all of these characteristics. Symptoms can also vary in intensity from person to person. Common TSC symptoms and indications include:

1. Skin Outward Signs:

• Facial angiofibromas are small, ruddy bumps or patches that appear on the nose and cheekbones most frequently.

• Hypomelanotic macules are light-colored skin regions.

• Shagreen patches are thick, elevated areas of skin that are commonly found on the lower back.

• Ungual fibromas are small, fleshy growths that develop around the fingernails or toenails.

• Forehead plaques are elevated, rough skin regions on the forehead.

2. Neurological Disorders:

• Seizures are a prevalent epileptic symptom that can vary in type and severity.

• Cognitive and developmental delays: Many TSC patients have learning disabilities, intellectual impairments, or developmental delays.

• Autism spectrum disorder (ASD): TSC is associated with an increased risk of ASD, as well as social and communication difficulties in some individuals.

3. Cognitive Engagement:

• Cortical tubers: Abnormal growths in the cortex (outer layer) of the brain that may result in neurological symptoms.

• Subependymal nodules (SENs) are small growths in the ventricles of the brain.

• Subependymal giant cell astrocytomas (SEGAs): Benign brain tumors that can induce blockages in the brain's fluid-filled spaces (hydrocephalus).

4. Kidney Participation:

• Renal angiomyolipomas: benign kidney tumors that can cause pain, hemorrhage, or impairment of kidney function.

5. Cardiac Participation:

• Cardiac rhabdomyomas: Heart tumors that are frequently diagnosed in infancy. They typically diminish and may eventually disappear.

6. Lung Impairment:

• Pulmonary lymphangioleiomyomatosis (LAM): Abnormal growth of smooth muscle cells in the lungs, which may cause respiratory difficulties.

7. Eye Malformations:

• Retinal hamartomas: benign retinal lesions that can impair vision.

• Other eye problems: TSC can lead to cataracts, glaucoma, and refractive defects, among others.

8. Additional Symptoms:

• Enamel pits: tiny fissures or cavities on the teeth.

• Liver involvement: TSC can infrequently cause liver hamartomas or lesions.

• Behavioral and psychiatric concerns: Some people with TSC may experience behavioral issues, anxiety, or mood disorders.

TSC can manifest in a variety of ways, with some patients experiencing only mild cutaneous manifestations and others experiencing more severe neurological or systemic complications.

Individuals with TSC require an early diagnosis and comprehensive medical care to effectively manage their condition and address their unique requirements. Treatment is often tailored to the individual's symptoms and may involve medications, surgery, or other interventions aimed at controlling seizures, managing tumors, and addressing developmental and behavioral challenges.

Diagnosis And Assessment

Tuberous sclerosis (TSC) is typically diagnosed and evaluated using a combination of clinical assessment, imaging investigations, and genetic testing. Due to the fact that TSC can affect multiple organs and systems, a multidisciplinary approach involving specialists from various medical disciplines is often required.

Here are the main components of the TSC evaluation and diagnosis process:

1. Clinical Evaluation:

• Medical History: The healthcare provider will collect a thorough medical history, including information about the patient's symptoms, developmental milestones, family history, and previous diagnoses and treatments.

• Physical Examination: A comprehensive physical examination will be performed to evaluate for characteristic skin findings, neurological symptoms, and other clinical characteristics associated with TSC.

2. Neurological Evaluation:

• Seizure Evaluation: If seizures are present, a comprehensive evaluation will be performed to ascertain their type and frequency. During seizures, electroencephalography (EEG) may be used to monitor brain activity.

• Developmental and Behavioral Evaluation: A developmental evaluation may be performed to evaluate cognitive and motor skills, as well as behavioral and social development.

3. Imaging Research:

• Brain Imaging: Magnetic resonance imaging (MRI) is typically used to detect the presence of cortical tubers, subependymal nodules (SENs), or subependymal giant cell astrocytomas (SEGAs) in the brain.

• Renal Imaging: Imaging investigations, such as ultrasound or MRI, can be used to assess the kidneys for renal angiomyolipomas.

• Cardiac Imaging: An echocardiogram (ultrasound of the heart) may be conducted to assess for cardiac rhabdomyomas.

4. Vision Examination:

• An ophthalmologist may conduct a comprehensive eye exam to detect retinal hamartomas and other eye abnormalities.

5. Testing Genetics:

• Genetic testing is essential for diagnosing TSC. It requires mutation analysis of the TSC1 and TSC2 genes. The identification of a pathogenic mutation in one of these genes confirms the diagnosis of Tuberous Sclerosis Complex.

• In cases where genetic testing does not disclose a mutation but clinical features strongly suggest TSC, additional testing may be necessary.

6. Skin Analysis:

• A dermatologist may evaluate a patient's skin for distinctive skin lesions, such as facial angiofibromas, hypomelanotic macules, shagreen patches, and ungual fibromas.

7. Other Assessments:

• Additional evaluations may be conducted based on the specific symptoms of the individual. This may include lung function tests for pulmonary involvement or dental examinations for pitted enamel.

8. Evaluation of the family and genetic counseling:

• If a person is diagnosed with TSC, genetic counseling is recommended to assess the risk of transmitting the condition to future generations and to offer support to affected individuals and their families.

The diagnosis of TSC can be complex due to the variable character of the disorder and the wide range of potential symptoms. A comprehensive evaluation, including genetic testing, is necessary for accurate diagnosis and to guide the development of appropriate management and treatment plans. Optimizing the welfare and quality of life of individuals with TSC requires an early diagnosis and intervention.

A group of healthcare professionals, such as neurologists, geneticists, dermatologists, and other specialists, may collaborate to provide comprehensive care and individualized management plans.

CHAPTER THREE
Administration And Treatment

The management and treatment of tuberous sclerosis (TSC) focuses on addressing the specific symptoms and complications that individuals may encounter.

Due to the fact that TSC can affect multiple organ systems, a multidisciplinary approach encompassing a number of specialists is frequently required to provide comprehensive care. Key aspects of

TSC management and treatment include.

1. Epilepsy Management:

• Antiepileptic Medications: Seizures are a prevalent symptom of TSC, and the choice of antiepileptic medications depends on the type and frequency of seizures. Typically, medications are prescribed to control and manage seizures.

2. Support for Neurodevelopment and Behavior:

• Early Intervention: Therapies and support for motor, speech, and cognitive development may be provided for children with developmental delays through early intervention programs.

• Behavioral Interventions: Behavioral therapy and interventions may be useful for addressing behavioral difficulties, particularly in individuals with autism spectrum disorder (ASD) or other behavioral issues.

3. Intervention and Surgery for Brain Tumors:

• Subependymal Giant Cell Astrocytomas (SEGAs): Surgical removal or intervention may be required if SEGAs cause symptoms or obstructions in the brain's fluid spaces (hydrocephalus).

• Other Brain Lesions: Depending on their location and impact on neurological function, surgical resection or other interventions may be considered for other brain lesions.

4. Kidney Participation:

• Renal Angiomyolipomas: These kidney tumors may be treated with embolization (blocking the blood vessels that supply the tumor), surgical removal, or medication to limit tumor growth.

5. Cardiac Administration:

- Cardiac Rhabdomyomas: These heart tumors diminish and resolve on their own in the majority of cases. However, monitoring by a pediatric cardiologist is essential to ensure proper heart function.

6. Pulmonary Administration:

- Pulmonary Lymphangioleiomyomatosis (LAM): If breathing difficulties develop, LAM may be treated with surveillance of lung function, medications, and oxygen therapy.

7. Ophthalmic Treatment:

• Routine eye exams are essential for monitoring and treating retinal hamartomas and other eye conditions. In some instances, therapy may be necessary.

8. Dental Health:

• Individuals with TSC should have routine dental examinations, and enamel defects can be treated as necessary.

9. Counseling for Genetic Considerations:

• Genetic counseling is recommended for individuals and families affected by TSC in order to assess the risk of transmitting the condition to future generations and to provide information and assistance for family planning.

10. Investigation and Clinical Tests:

• Some individuals with TSC may be eligible to participate in clinical trials and research studies, particularly if novel therapies or interventions are being investigated.

11. Psychosocial Assistance:

• TSC can significantly affect the emotional and psychological health of affected individuals and their families. Groups of support, counseling, and other resources for grappling with and managing stress can be beneficial.

The management of TSC is highly individualized, and treatment plans are tailored to the specific requirements and symptoms of each person.

Regular follow-up appointments with healthcare providers, including specialists, are necessary to monitor the condition's progression and modify treatment plans as needed. Research and treatment options advancements continue to enhance the care and outcomes for TSC patients.

Surgical interventions may be considered as part of the management of tuberous sclerosis (TSC) when certain symptoms or complications require medical intervention. The decision to undergo surgery and the specific surgical procedures depend on the condition and organs or systems of the individual.

Here are some frequent surgical interventions associated with TSC:

1. Removal of Brain Tumors:

• Subependymal Giant Cell Astrocytomas (SEGAs): Surgical resection is often required when

SEGAs grow large enough to induce symptoms or blockages in the brain's fluid spaces (hydrocephalus). This procedure involves the removal of the tumor or the release of the obstruction.

2. Management of Renal Angiomyolipoma (AML):

• Embolization: Large or symptomatic renal AMLs may be candidates for embolization. In this procedure, the blood vessels that supply the tumor are occluded, thereby reducing the risk of hemorrhage or rupture.

• Surgical Resection: In some cases, particularly if embolization is ineffective or if the AML is causing severe kidney injury, the tumor may be surgically removed.

3. Skin Lesion Excision:

• Dermatologic Procedures: TSC-related facial angiofibromas and other skin lesions can be cosmetically bothersome. To eradicate or diminish the appearance of these skin lesions, dermatological procedures such as laser therapy and surgical excision may be utilized.

4. Heart Surgery:

• In rare instances where cardiac rhabdomyomas cause substantial heart-related issues, cardiac surgery may be considered to remove or treat the tumors. However, these tumors frequently disappear on their own over time.

5. Lung Operations:

• Pulmonary Lymphangioleiomyomatosis (LAM): Although rare, severe cases of LAM may necessitate lung transplantation. When lung function is severely impaired and other treatments have failed, lung transplantation may be considered.

6. Therapy for Epilepsy:

• Individuals with TSC who have medically refractory epilepsy (seizures that do not respond to medications) may be candidates for epilepsy surgery or vagus nerve stimulator (VNS) implantation.

7. TSC is sometimes associated with skeletal abnormalities or scoliosis. To correct these issues and enhance mobility and comfort, orthopedic surgery may be required.

8. Dental Treatments:

• Enamel Pits: Dental procedures, such as fillings or sealants, can be used to treat enamel pits, a common dental symptom of TSC.

9. Eye Operations:

• Retinal Hamartomas: Surgical removal or other ophthalmic procedures may be considered in cases where retinal hamartomas significantly impair vision.

Notably, surgical interventions are typically contemplated when the benefits outweigh the risks, and the decision is made case by case. A team of healthcare professionals, including specialists in neurosurgery, urology, dermatology, cardiology, and other relevant disciplines, determines the approach and timing of surgery.

Prior to undergoing any surgical procedure, patients and their families should have a thorough discussion with their healthcare team about the potential risks, benefits, and expected outcomes. Surgical interventions are frequently a component of a comprehensive treatment plan that also includes ongoing medical management and therapies to address the various aspects of TSC.

CHAPTER FOUR
Adaptation And Support

Tuberous sclerosis (TSC) can affect a variety of aspects of life, including physical health, cognitive development, and emotional well-being, making it difficult for individuals with the condition and their families to cope. Individuals and families coping with TSC can utilize the following strategies and sources of support:

1. Care and Monitoring Medical:

• Attend medical consultations with specialists who have experience treating TSC on a regular basis.

• Maintain an open line of communication with healthcare providers in order to address concerns and monitor progress.

2. Education and Knowledge:

• Acquire as much information as possible regarding TSC, its symptoms, and available treatments.

• Consult credible information sources, such as TSC-specific organizations and medical resources.

3. Assistance Groups:

• Participate in online and offline TSC support groups and communities. These communities provide a forum for connecting with others who face comparable obstacles.

• Share experiences, ask questions, and acquire insight from individuals with direct experience with TSC.

4. Counseling and Counseling:

• Consider individual or family counseling to address the emotional and psychological aspects of living with TSC.

• Behavioral therapy and interventions may be useful for addressing behavioral difficulties in TSC patients.

5. Awareness and Advocacy:

• Advocate for your educational demands or those of your child. Collaborate with educators to develop an Individualized Education Program (IEP) or a 504 Plan in order to provide appropriate school accommodations and support.

• Raise community awareness about TSC and advocate for TSC research and funding.

6. Services for Respite Care and Support:

• Seek out respite care services to provide temporary reprieve for primary caregivers and to ensure that individuals with TSC receive the necessary care and attention.

• Investigate support services, such as home healthcare and in-home therapies, to help with daily duties and therapies.

7. Legal and Financial Planning:

• Consider financial planning to account for the prospective long-term costs of managing medical needs and therapies associated with TSC.

• Establish legal provisions, if necessary, such as guardianship or power of attorney.

8. Personal care:

• Caregivers should prioritize self-care in order to avoid exhaustion and preserve their physical and mental health.

• Make time for relaxation, exercise, pastimes, and enjoyable activities.

9. Counseling for Genetic Considerations:

• Consider genetic counseling if you have or are a carrier for Tay-Sachs disease in order to assess the risk of transmitting the condition on to future generations and make informed family planning decisions.

10. Advocacy and Participation in Research:

• Consider participating in TSC-related research studies or clinical trials in order to advance prospective treatments and knowledge.

• Advocate for research and awareness initiatives to receive funding and support.

11. Peer guidance:

• Communicate with families who have been affected by TSC for an extended period of time. They can offer advice and assistance based on their experiences.

12. Celebrate Achievements:

• Commemorate small and large accomplishments and milestones, whether they pertain to medical advancements, educational achievements, or personal objectives.

Remember that every person with TSC is unique, with varying requirements and experiences. Finding a supportive community and gaining access to situation-specific resources can be of great assistance in overcoming the challenges of TSC.

In addition, keeping abreast of new developments in research and treatment options can offer hope and possibilities for enhanced care and quality of life.

Educational And Developing Difficulties

Due to the broad range of neurological and cognitive manifestations associated with tuberous sclerosis (TSC), educational and developmental difficulties are common in individuals with this condition.

The severity of these obstacles can differ from person to person. Listed below are some of the most common educational and developmental obstacles faced by individuals with TSC, as well as strategies and considerations for overcoming them:

1. Delay in the Developmental Process:

• Many individuals with TSC experience developmental delays in walking, communicating, and social interaction.

• Early intervention services, which may include physical therapy, speech therapy, and occupational therapy, can assist in addressing these delays and fostering development.

2. Cognitive Deficits:

• Certain individuals with TSC may exhibit cognitive impairments, including intellectual disabilities.

• Individualized education plans (IEPs) or 504 Plans in educational contexts can provide individualized academic support and accommodations for students with TSC.

3. Behavioral Difficulties:

• Certain individuals with TSC may display challenging behaviors, such as impulsivity, aggression, or difficulties with emotional regulation.

• Behavioral therapy and interventions can be effective in managing and decreasing problem behaviors. Positive reinforcement and structured routines may also prove beneficial.

4. Spectrum Disorders of Autism (ASD):

• TSC is associated with an increased risk for ASD, and some individuals may be diagnosed with both TSC and ASD.

• Early diagnosis, early intervention services, and applied behavior analysis (ABA) therapy can facilitate the development of communication and social skills in individuals with ASD.

5. Seizures:

• Seizures are a prevalent symptom of TSC and can impair cognitive and learning abilities.

• Appropriate seizure management with antiepileptic drugs is necessary to mitigate the impact of seizures on academic progress.

6. Attention and Executive Performance:

• Some individuals with TSC may struggle with executive functions such as planning, organization, and impulse control.

• Educational accommodations such as extended testing time, a distraction-free environment, and assistance with organization can be advantageous.

7. IEPs: Individualized Education Plans

• Collaborate with educators and specialists to develop and implement individualized education programs (IEPs) that are tailored to the specific requirements of students with TSC.

• Individualized Education Programs (IEPs) may include academic, behavioral, and social development objectives, as well as accommodations and services.

8. Social Competence Development:

• Social skills deficits are common in individuals with TSC, particularly those with ASD.

• Social skills training and opportunities for social interaction, such as group activities and organizations, can aid in the development of social competence.

9. Routine Observation and Communication:

• Maintain open communication between parents, educators, and healthcare providers to ensure that the individual's educational and developmental requirements are being met.

• It is crucial to monitor progress frequently and modify interventions as necessary.

10. Transition Preparation:

• Transition planning becomes essential as individuals with TSC approach adolescence and maturity. This includes preparation for higher education, employment, and independent living.

11. Advocate for your child's educational requirements and rights, ensuring that he or she receives the necessary support and accommodations in school.

It is essential to emphasize that individuals with TSC have unique strengths and abilities, and that, with the right support and interventions, they can make significant educational and developmental gains.

Early diagnosis, early intervention services, and a network of supportive and well-informed caregivers, educators, and healthcare professionals are crucial in assisting individuals with TSC to realize their full potential.

Summary And Prognosis

Tuberous sclerosis (TSC) is a genetic disorder characterized by the development of benign lesions in multiple organs and body systems. It is caused by mutations in the TSC1 or TSC2 genes and can affect the epidermis, brain, kidneys, heart, lungs, and eyes, among other organs. TSC is a rare disorder with a variable clinical presentation, and its diagnosis frequently involves clinical evaluation, imaging investigations, and genetic analysis.

Management and treatment of TSC are multidisciplinary and individualized according to the requirements of each patient. Medication to control seizures, surgical interventions to address tumors or obstructions, therapies to manage developmental and behavioral challenges, and ongoing medical monitoring may be employed as treatment strategies.

Accessing resources, support groups, and services that address the medical, educational, and emotional aspects of the condition is necessary for coping with TSC and providing assistance to affected individuals. Improving the quality of life for individuals with TSC and their families requires early intervention, advocacy, and a supportive community.

In the future, ongoing research and advances in genetics and medical remedies offer hope for improved management and outcomes for those affected by TSC.

As knowledge and therapies advance, TSC patients and their families can anticipate more effective treatments and enhanced support systems to meet the disorder's unique challenges.

THE END

69